Low Calorie Steam Cookbook

Healthy Steam Recipes That are Hassle-Free & Delicious

Table of Contents

Introduction

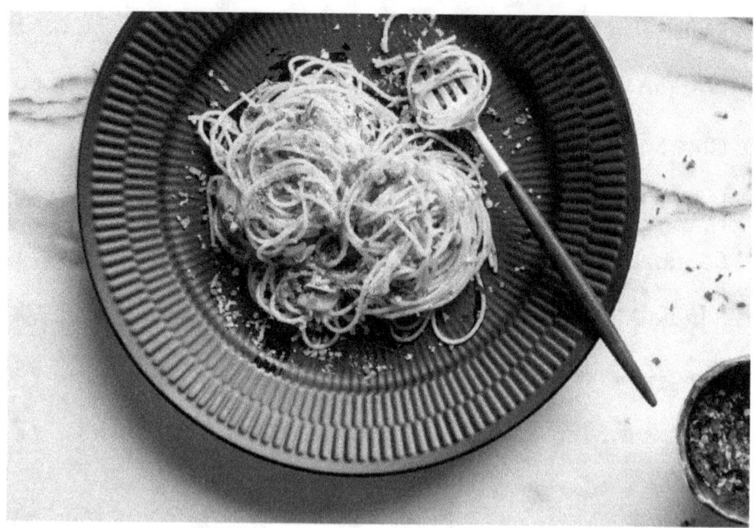

Steaming has been a method of cooking for a few years now, this is because steaming is more versatile, healthy and is a simpler way of cooking. The method of steaming is the ideal choice for people who are seeking or are on a controlled low-calorie diet.

Low Calorie Steam Cookbook is designed to provide 30 healthy and nutritious recipes containing meals that fall between 300-500 calories perfect for a low-calorie controlled diet. Each unique recipe makes two servings and have been cooked and tested for its caloric value and serving. This magnificent cookbook is sectioned with a collection of healthy, nutritious and delicious seafood, poultry and meat dishes.

Chinese Ground Beef

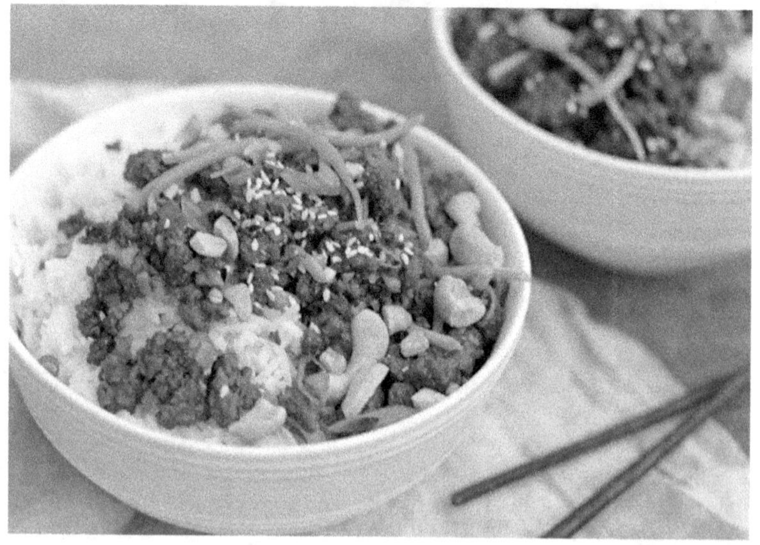

This delicious Chinese ground beef recipe will leave your taste buds tingling.

Serves: 2

Time: 40 mins.

Calories per serving: 490

Ingredients:

- Rice (3 ½ oz, long grain)
- Water (1 cup, boiling)

- Salt (large pinch)
- Beef (9 oz, ground)
- Ginger (1 tsp, grated)
- Soy sauce (2 tsp)
- Egg (1)
- Garlic (1 clove, crushed)
- Hoisin sauce (1 tbsp)
- Scallions (chopped)
- Salt & pepper to taste

Directions:

1. Combine the boiling water, rice and salt in a glass bowl (steam-proof) and place in the second tier of the steamer.

2. Next, cover steamer with the lid and steam for approximately 10 minutes.

3. When finished, mix together the ginger, ground beef, soy sauce, egg and crushed garlic using your hands.

4. Form into two meat patties and use hoisin sauce to brush then place in the bottom tier of steamer.

5. Cover steamer with lid and steam for an additional 20 minutes until rice becomes tender and the beef is thoroughly cooked.

6. Arrange ground beef on a plate and use scallions to sprinkle and serve.

Steamed Beef & Basil Meatballs

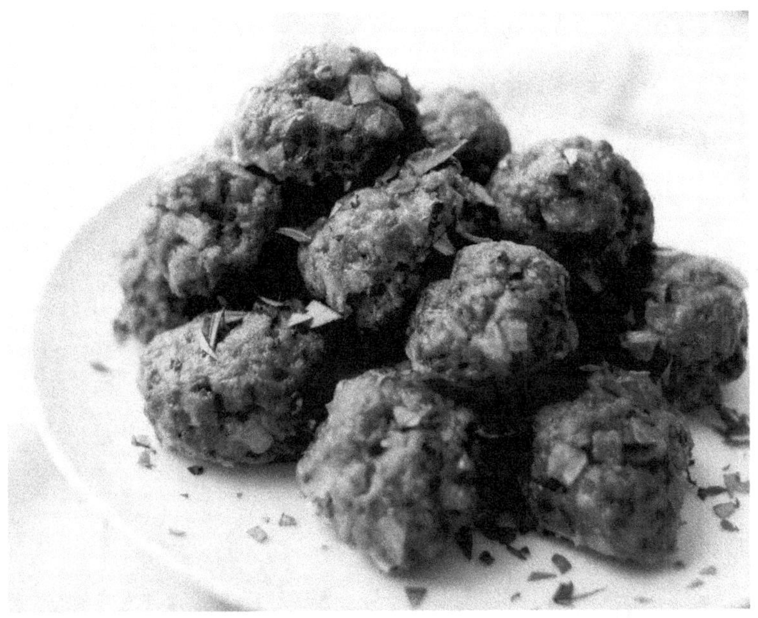

Steamed Beef and Basil Meatballs are certainly no stranger at the dinner table.

Serves: 2

Time: 30-40 mins.

Calories per serving: 490

Ingredients:

- Rice (3 ½ oz, long grain)
- Water (1 cup, boiling)
- Salt (large pinch)
- Beef (9 oz, ground)
- Worcestershire sauce (1 tbsp)
- Egg (1)
- Basil (1 bunch, fresh, chopped, few leaves for garnish)
- Garlic (1 clove, crushed)
- Salt pepper to taste

Directions:

1. Combine the boiling water, rice, and salt in a glass bowl (steam proof) and place in the second tier of steamer.

2. Cover steamer with lid and steam for approxiamtely10 minutes.

3. Next, mix together the ground beef, Worcestershire sauce, basil, egg and garlic using hands.

4. Form mixture into 10 meatballs (small) and place meatballs into the bottom tier of steamer.

5. Place lid over the steamer and steam for an additional 10-20 minutes, until rice becomes tender and meatballs are thoroughly cooked.

6. When finished, serve rice in a shallow bowl with meatballs piled on top, use reserved basil to sprinkle.

Bratwurst Steamed Cabbage

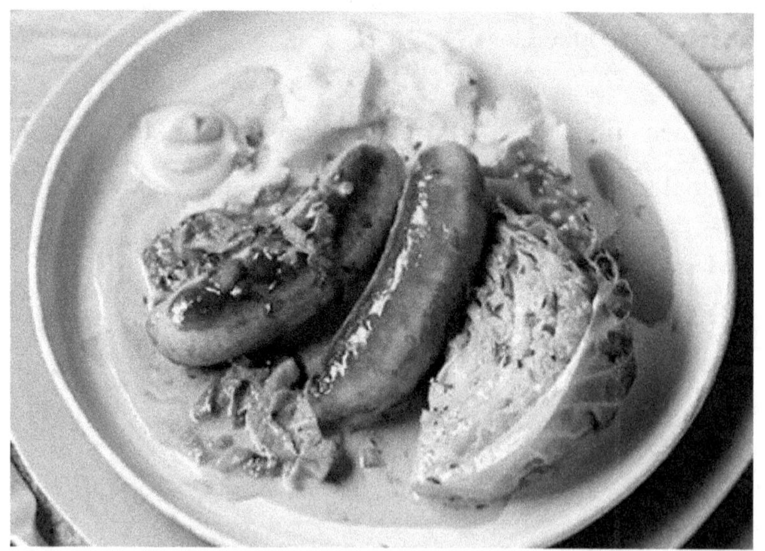

This recipe is utilizing bratwurst to the fullest combining it with healthy and delicious steamed cabbage.

Serves: 2

Time: 25 mins.

Calories per serving: 495

Ingredients:

- Bratwurst sausage (9 oz)
- Butter spread (1 tbsp, low fat)

- Garlic (1 clove, crushed)
- Cabbage (1, green pointed, shredded)
- Cheese (1 tbsp, parmesan)
- Salt pepper to taste

Directions:

1. First step Is to place bratwurst sausage in bottom tier of steamer.

2. Next add the garlic and butter to a ramekin dish and tightly cover with aluminum foil.

3. Place mixture and cabbage (shredded) in the second tier of steamer.

4. Place lid over steamer and cover then cook for approximately 10-15 minutes, until sausages are thoroughly cooked, and the cabbage becomes tender.

5. Remove sausages and cut into diagonal thick slices and toss the garlic butter with the shredded cabbage and evenly arrange in a bowl (shallow).

6. Place sausage on top and use parmesan cheese and black pepper to sprinkle.

Steamed Thai Fish Fillets

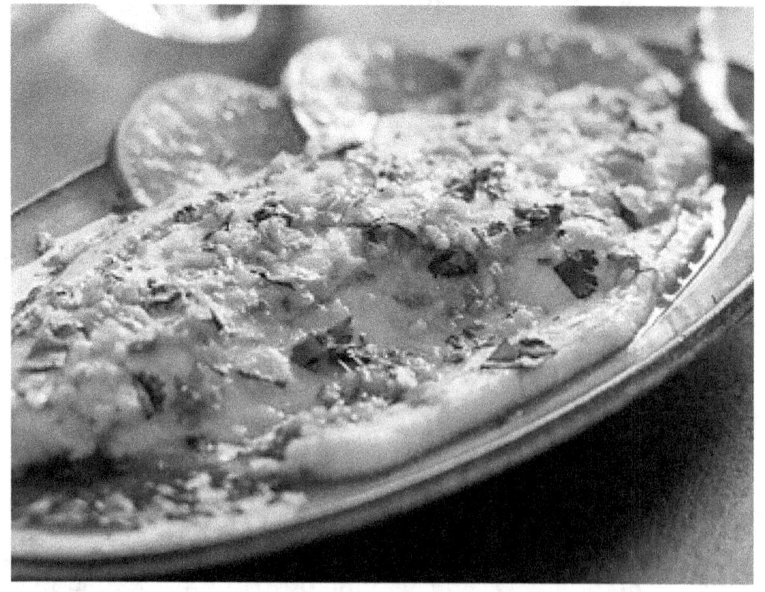

Simple and delicious steamed Thai Fish Fillets, sure to leave you speechless.

Serves: 2

Time: 35 mins.

Calories per serving: 240

Ingredients:

- Fish fillets (2, firm, white, 6oz)
- Cayenne pepper (1/2 tsp)
- Ginger (1 tsp, freshly grated)
- Garlic (1 clove, crushed)
- Lime juice (2 tbsp)
- Soy sauce (2 tbsp)
- Sugar (1/2 tsp, brown)
- Cabbage (2, small, Chinese, shredded)
- Salt pepper (to taste)
- Lime (1, zest)

Directions:

1. Mix the ginger, cayenne pepper, garlic, lime juice, lime zest, soy sauce sugar together in a large bowl.

2. Next add the cabbage (shredded) and thoroughly combine.

3. Evenly arrange fish fillets on a large piece of aluminum foil. Season fish and scatter the cabbage (shredded) marinade on top.

4. Fold aluminum into a parcel around the fillets leaving adequate room so that steam can freely circulate around the sides and top of fish fillets.

5. Place fillets into the bottom tier of steamer and cover with the lid and steam for approximately 15 minutes, until the fillets are thoroughly cooked, and the cabbage is tender.

6. Evenly arrange on a suitable sized plate. Season and serve. Enjoy.

Steamed Scallop Salad

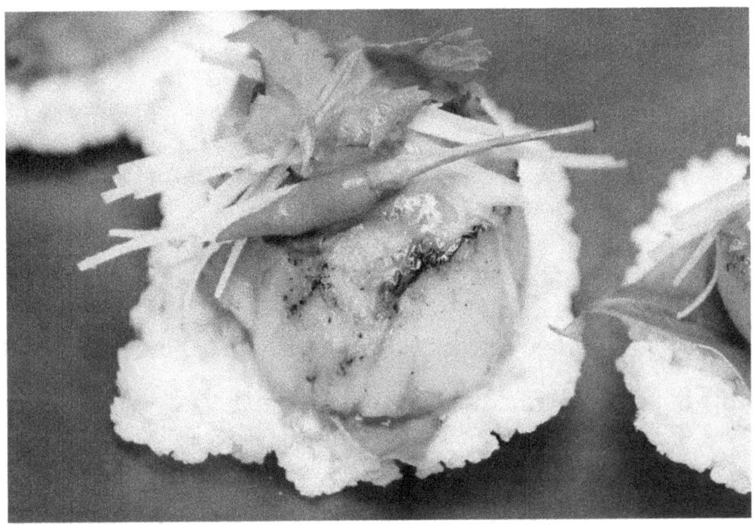

A healthy steamy salad recipe that will leave a smile on your face.

Serves: 2

Time: 15 mins.

Calories per serving: 170

Ingredients:

- Scallops (8, shelled, cleaned)
- Soy sauce (2 tbsp)
- Honey (2 tsp, clear)

- Chili flakes (½ tsp, crushed)
- Lime juice (1 tbsp)
- Ginger (1 tsp, freshly grated)
- Salad leaves (7oz, mixed)
- Salt pepper (to taste)

Directions:

1. In a suitable size bowl, combine soy sauce, ginger, honey, chili flakes, and lime juice together to make a dressing.

2. Next step is to toss scallops with the dressing until coated well. Reserve any leftover dressing.

3. Place scallops in the bottom tier of steamer and use the lid to cover.

4. Steam for a minimum of 5 minutes, until thoroughly cooked.

5. Serve on a bed of salad leaves (mixed) with the remaining dressing over the top.

Balsamic Tuna Steak Rice

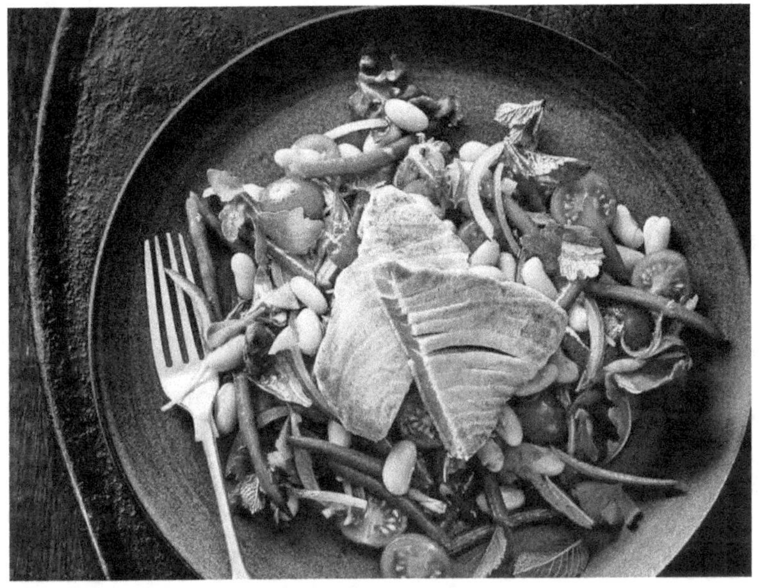

A unique delicious recipe prepared in less than an hour.

Serves: 2

Time: 42 mins.

Calories per serving: 470

Ingredients:

- Rice (3½ oz, long grain)
- vegetable stock (1 cup, hot)

- tuna steaks (2, fresh, 5oz)

- balsamic vinegar (3 tbsp)

- garlic (1, crushed)

- soy sauce (2 tbsp)

- Salt pepper (to taste)

Directions:

1. In a glass bowl (steam proof) combine the rice and vegetable stock and place in the second tier of steamer.

2. Use the lid to cover steamer and steam for approximately 20 minutes.

3. Season the tuna steaks and mix together the garlic, balsamic vinegar and soy sauce in a ramekin dish (small).

4. Cover with aluminum foil and place on the bottom tier of steamer alongside the tuna steaks (seasoned).

5. Cover with lid and steam for an additional 12 minutes, until tuna is thoroughly cooked, and rice becomes tender.

6. Serve tuna steaks on a bed of rice with the balsamic sauce poured over the top.

Oyster Sauce Fish Broccolini

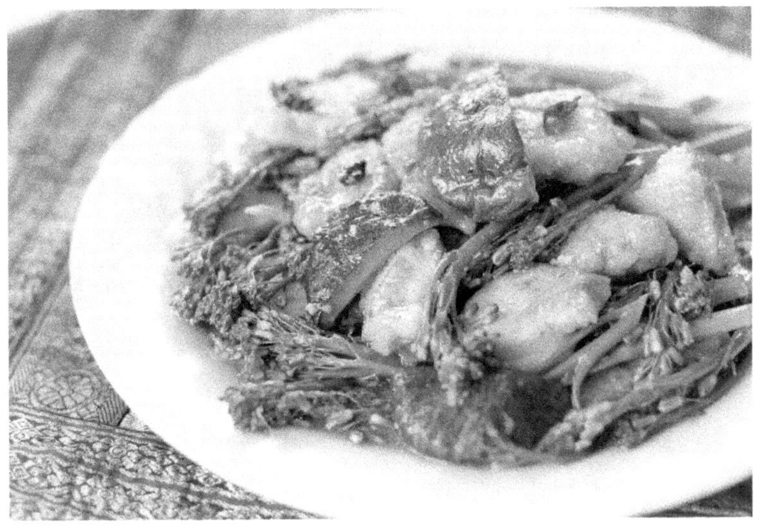

This scrumptious Oyster Sauce Fish Broccolini is prepared quickly and is the ideal healthy choice for lunch.

Serves: 2

Time: 25 mins.

Calories per serving: 290

Ingredients:

- Fish fillets (2, firm, white, 6 oz)
- Ginger (1 tsp, freshly grated)
- Garlic clove (1, crushed)

- Oyster sauce (2 tbsp)
- Soy sauce (2 tbsp)
- Broccoli (9 oz, tender stem)
- Salt pepper (to taste)

Directions:

1. Mix together the ginger, garlic clove, oyster sauce, soy sauce in a bowl to form a marinade.

2. Next step is to place the fish fillets on a large piece of aluminum foil and use a little marinade to brush.

3. Add broccoli to the bowl with the remainder of marinade and combine well.

4. Tip this mixture over the fish and fold aluminum into a parcel leaving Fold aluminum into a parcel around the fillets leaving adequate room so that steam can freely circulate around the sides and top of broccoli.

5. When finished, place in the bottom tier of steamer and use lid to cover. Steam for approximately 15 minutes, until fish is thoroughly cooked, and broccoli becomes tender.

6. Evenly arrange on a plate. Season and serve. Enjoy.

Sliced Chicken Chickpea Salad

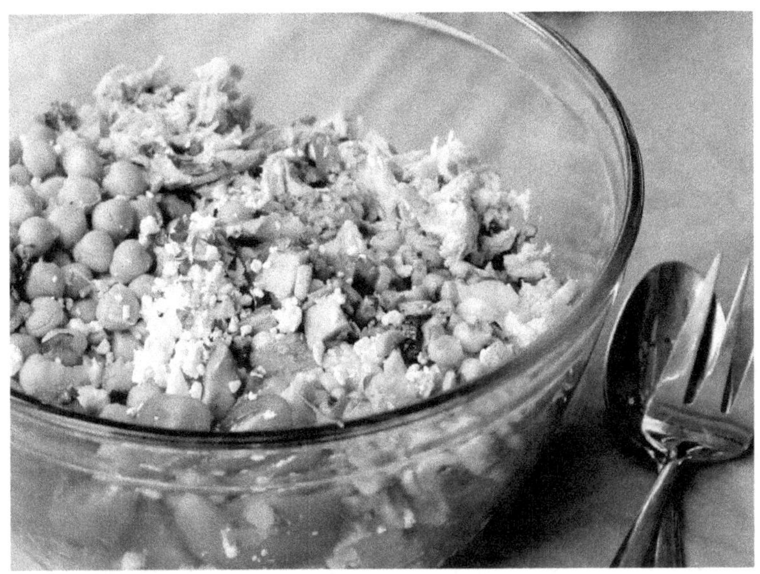

This delicious recipe is a well-known combination known for its high protein properties containing only 440 calories.

Serves: 2

Time: 30 mins.

Calories per serving: 440

Ingredients:

- Chicken breasts (2, 4 oz)
- Cider (4 tbsp, dry)

- Mustard (4 tbsp, dry)
- Honey (1 tbsp)
- Chickpeas (7oz, tinned, drained)
- Rocket (7 oz)
- Lemon juice (2 tsp)
- Cream (4 tbsp, low fat)
- Salt pepper (to taste)

Directions:

1. First step is to season the chicken and combine with the honey, cider and mustard together in a large ramekin dish and use a piece of aluminum to cover.

2. When finished, place the ramekin dish into the bottom tier of steamer.

3. Use lid to cover and steam for approximately 20 minutes, until chicken is thoroughly cooked.

4. Toss the rocket, lemon juice, chickpeas together and slice the chicken into thick slices.

5. Lay on top of the chickpeas and rocket and stir the cream through the honey (warm) in the large ramekin dish and pour over chicken salad.

Steamed Oyster Sauce Steak

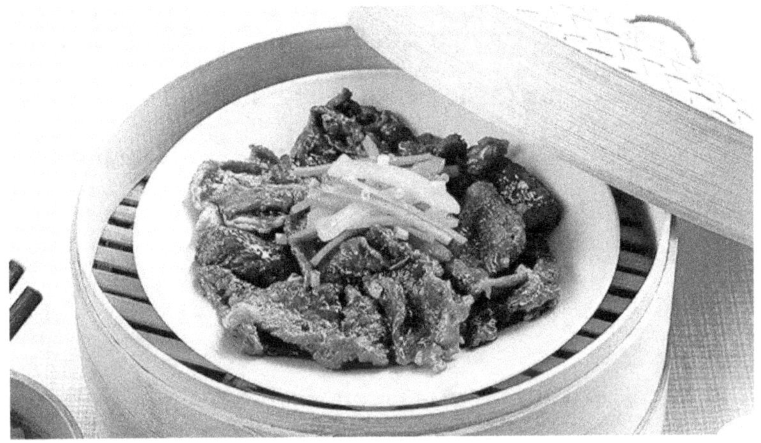

Convenient and tasty, an easy to follow recipe, enriched with oyster sauce.

Serves: 2

Time: 25 mins.

Calories per serving: 340

Ingredients:

- Oyster sauce (3 tbsp)
- Salt brown sugar (½ tsp each)
- Soy sauce (1 tsp)
- Garlic clove (1, crushed)

- Sirloin steak (9 oz trimmed, cut into strips)
- Bok choy (quartered)
- Carrots (2, cut into batons)
- Red pepper (1, deseeded finely sliced)
- Spring onions (1 bunch /scallions, sliced lengthways)
- Salt pepper (to taste)

Directions:

1. In a bowl (steam-proof) combine the oyster sauce, sugar, salt, soy sauce and garlic to create a marinade.

2. Add the steak (sliced) to the bowl, mix thoroughly then place in steamer in the bottom tier.

3. Put the carrots, bok choy and peppers in the steamer in the second tier and cook for approximately 10 minutes or until the steak is cooked to your preference and the vegetables are tender.

4. Join the vegetables and the steak together and serve in a bowl (shallow). Use the spring onions to sprinkle.

Pesto Penne Chicken

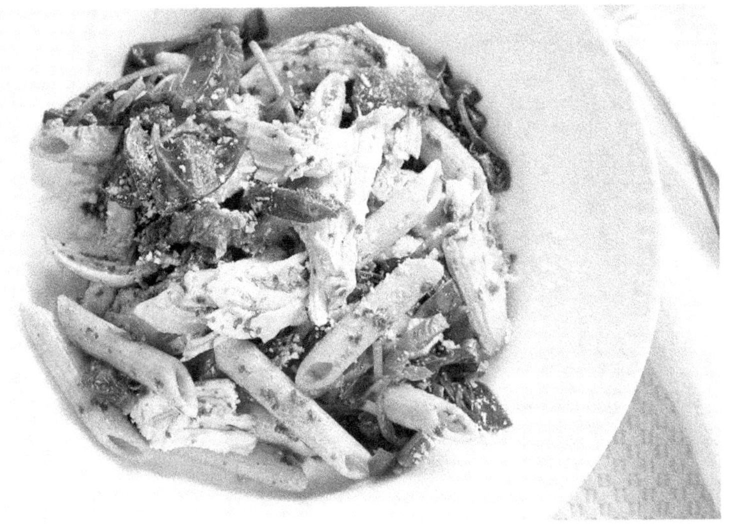

A delicious and healthy steaming hot Pesto Penne Chicken. Great meal if you are in a hurry.

Serves: 2

Time: 35 mins.

Calories per serving: 498

Ingredients:

- Garlic clove (1, crushed)
- Lemon juice (1 tbsp)

- Basil (1 tsp dried)

- Penne (5 oz)

- Chicken breasts (2, 4 oz)

- Pesto sauce (2 tbsp, green)

- Salt pepper (to taste)

Directions:

1. Mix the lemon juice, garlic basil and use this mixture to brush on to the chicken breasts.

2. Put the chicken in the bottom tier of the steamer and allow to cook for approximately 10 minutes.

3. Put the pasta in a glass bowl (steam-proof), cover with boiling water and add some salt (pinch).

4. Put in the second tier of the steamer, cover the lid and steam for an additional 10-15 minutes until the pasta becomes soft and tender and the chicken is cooked thoroughly.

5. Put in the second tier of the steamer, cover the lid and steam for an additional 10-15 minutes, until pasta becomes soft and tender and the chicken is cooked thoroughly.

6. Take out the chicken and cut each breast into slices (thick). Drain the pasta then mix well with the pesto sauce.

7. Serve the pesto penne in bowls (shallow) with the chicken breast arranged on the top.

Garlic Butter Chive Corn

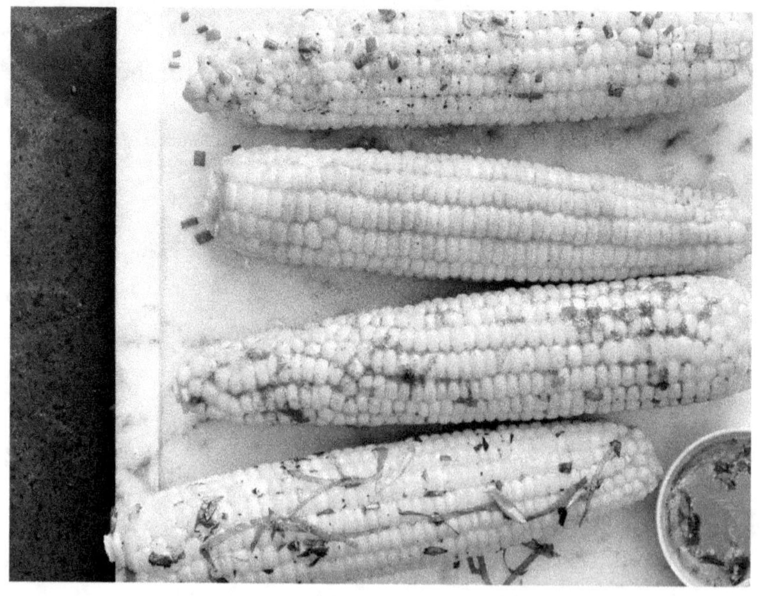

Garlic butter and chive, the perfect complement for fresh corn.

Serves: 2

Time: 35 mins.

Calories per serving: 170

Ingredients:

- Corn on the cob (2 fresh, medium)
- Butter (low fat, 1 oz, spread)
- Garlic cloves (2, crushed)
- Chives (1 tbsp, freshly chopped)
- Salt pepper (to taste)

Directions:

1. Take off the silky husks from the corn.

2. Put the cobs into the bottom tier of the steamer, cover with the lid and steam for approximately 10 minutes.

3. Add the butter, garlic and chives to a ramekin dish, cover tightly with foil and place on a tier above the steaming corn.

4. Cover the steamer again using the lid and continue to steam the corn for an additional 10-20 minutes or until the corn is cooked.

5. Remove the corn when it is tender and brush with the garlic butter. Season well and serve. Enjoy.

Smoked Sausage Dinner

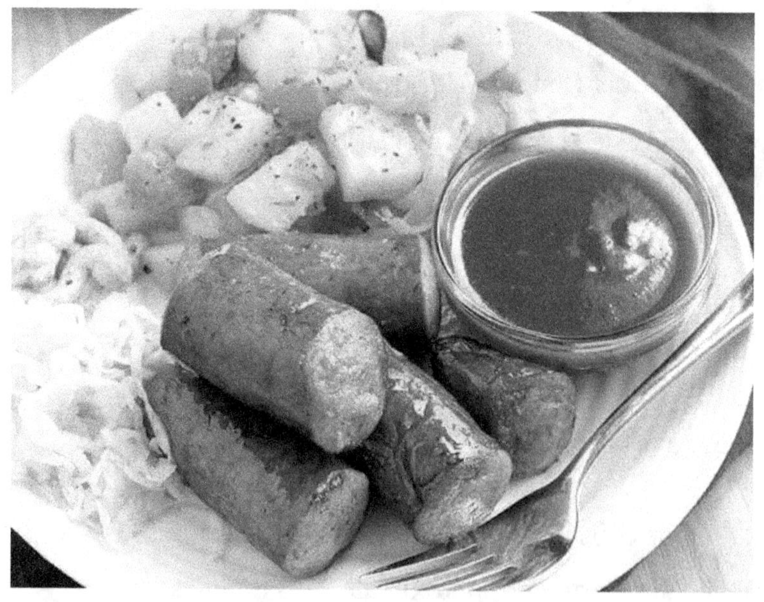

This super easy Smoked Sausage Dinner is a perfect weeknight dinner idea.

Serves: 2

Time: 25 mins.

Calories per serving: 490

Ingredients:

- Penne (5oz)
- Smoked sausage (7oz, low fat)
- Worcestershire sauce (1 tsp)
- Tomato passata/sauce (1 cup)
- Tomato puree/paste (1 tbsp)
- Salt brown sugar (½ tsp each)
- Garlic clove (1, peeled)
- Salt pepper (to taste)

Directions:

1. Put the pasta in a bowl (steam proof), cover with boiling water and some salt (a pinch). Put in the steamer in the bottom tier with the smoked sausage.

2. Add the Worcestershire sauce, passata, puree, salt sugar to a separate steam-proof bowl and combine well. Cover with foil tightly and put in the steamer in the second tier. Place the garlic clove next to it.

3. Use the lid to cover the steamer and cook for approximately 10-15 minutes

4. Crush the garlic then mix with the tomato sauce. Drain the pasta and cut the sausages into thick slices. Mix well.

5. Combine everything together thoroughly, check the sauce seasoning and serve as soon as finished.

Lamb Mint Couscous

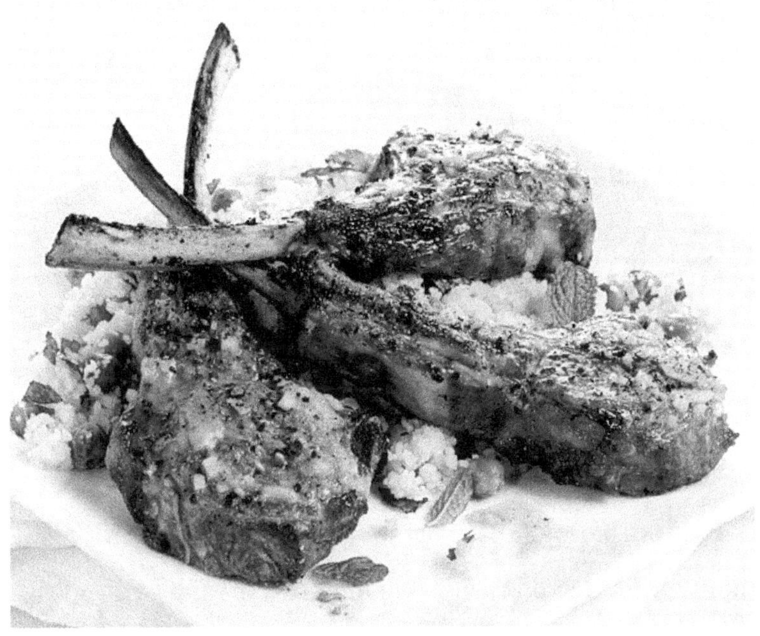

An aromatic tasty meal, the perfect way to use up lamb leftovers.

Serves: 2

Time: 30 mins.

Calories per serving: 470

Ingredients:

- Lamb steaks (2, lean, 4 oz)
- Garlic clove (1, crushed)
- Olive oil (1 tsp)
- Mint (2 tbsp, freshly chopped)
- Couscous (3½ oz)
- Vegetable stock (¾ cup hot)
- Salt pepper (to taste)

Directions:

1. First step is to place lamb steaks on a large piece of aluminum foil and brush using the olive oil and garlic.

2. Fold the aluminum into a parcel leaving adequate room for steam to freely circulate around the sides and top of the lamb.

3. Place lamb into the bottom tier of steamer use lid to cover. Cook for approximately 10 minutes.

4. When time has elapsed place the vegetable stock and couscous in a glass bowl (steam-proof) and stir once. Place in the second tier of steamer.

5. Cover with lid and steam for an additional 10 minutes, until the lamb is thoroughly cooked.

6. When finished, thoroughly fluff up couscous using a fork, and toss the mint (chopped) through it.

7. Serve lamb steaks with the couscous (minced) on the side. Season and serve. Enjoy.

Pork Prawn Dumplings

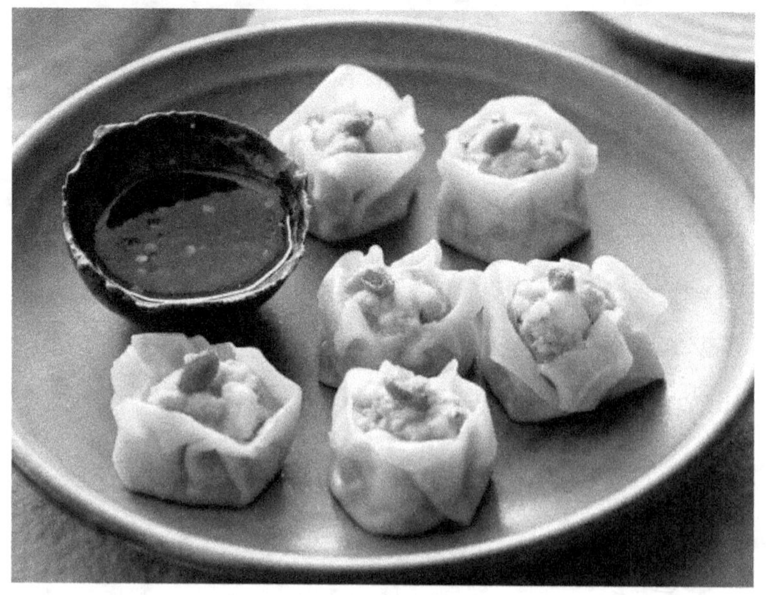

Pork and Prawn Dumplings, low-fat, impressive and delicious.

Serves: 2

Time: 22 mins.

Calories per serving: 360

Ingredients:

- Mince pork/ground pork (4 oz, lean)
- Prawns/shrimp (4 oz, raw)
- Soy sauce (1 tbsp)
- Fish sauce (1 tbsp)
- Ground ginger (½ tsp)
- Corn flour/cornstarch (1 tsp)
- Wonton dumpling wrappers (10-12)
- Plum sauce (2 tbsp)
- Salt pepper (to taste)

Directions:

1. In a food processer, place all the ingredients with exception of the plum sauce and the dumpling wrappers, into a food processor.

2. Blend until everything is well fused.

3. Lay the wonton wrappers out and in the center of each paper place 2 teaspoons of the pork mixture.

4. Take up both sides and put together to form a closed packet.

5. Place dumplings in the steamer in the bottom tier. Use the lid to cover and steam for approximately 12 minutes or until the dumplings are cooked.

6. Serve with plum sauce. Enjoy.

Eggs Ham Snack

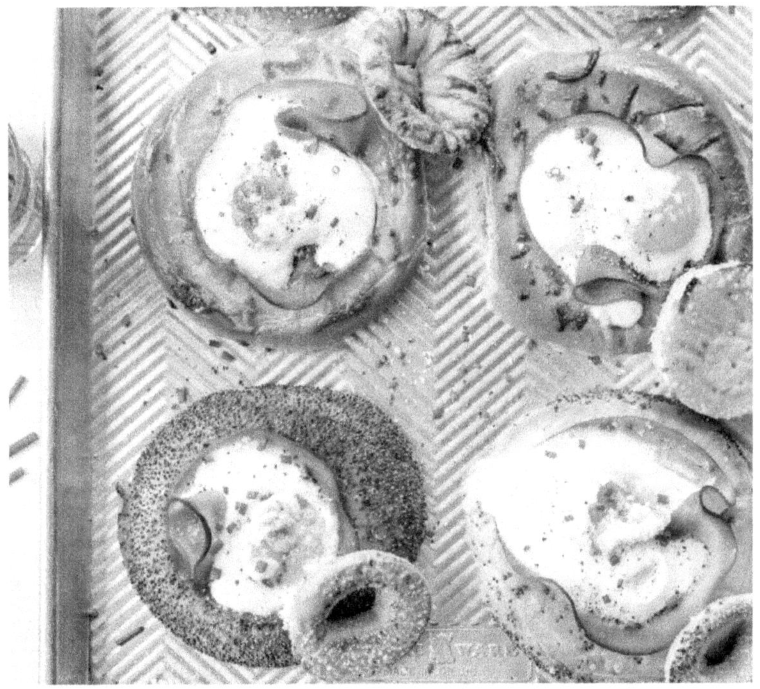

This egg and ham snack is delicious and easy to prepare.

Serves: 2

Time: 25 mins.

Calories per serving: 190

Ingredients:

- Eggs (4)
- Smoked ham (2 slices, lean, chopped)
- Tomato puree (2 tsp, sundried)
- Salt pepper (to taste)

Directions:

1. Put all the ingredients together.

2. Separate the mixture equally between two ramekin dishes (greased).

3. Place in the steamer on the bottom tier. Use the lid to cover steamer and steam for approximately 15-20 minutes.

Spiced Chicken Rice

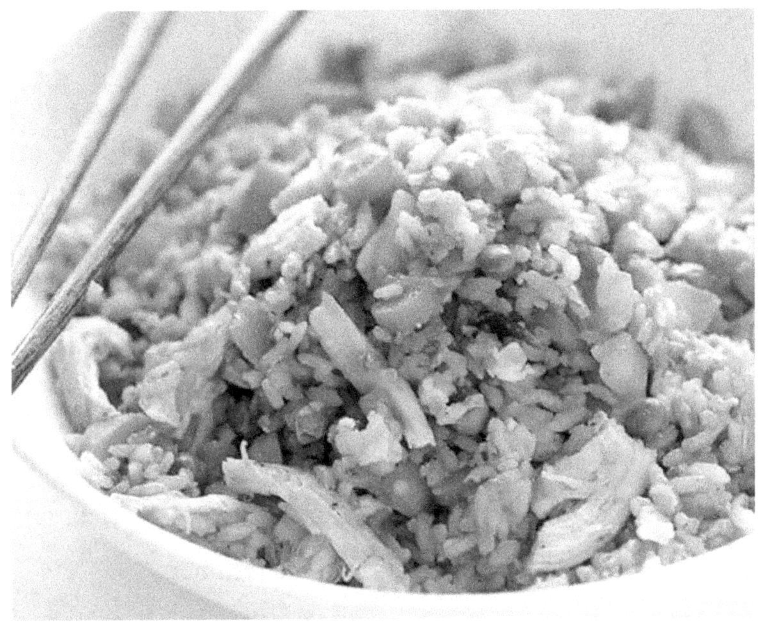

Nutritious, creamy and packed with flavor.

Serves: 2

Time: 45 mins.

Calories per serving: 420

Ingredients:

- Rice (3½ oz, long grain)
- Boiling water (1 cup)

- Salt (Large pinch)
- Saffron threads (Large pinch)
- Sultanas (2 tbsp, chopped)
- Chicken breasts (2 ,4 oz)
- Mango chutney (2 tbsp)
- Salt pepper (to taste)
- Ground cilantro/ coriander, cumin, cayenne pepper and turmeric (1/2 tsp)

Directions:

1. In a glass bowl (steam proof) combine the water, rice, salt saffron and put in the second tier of the steamer.

2. Use the lid to cover steamer then steam for approximately 10 minutes.

3. While waiting, mix the dried spices and coat the chicken breasts together in these.

4. Place the chicken in the steamer in the bottom tier and add the sultanas (chopped) to the rice.

5. Use the lid to cover the steamer and steam for approximately 20-25 minutes.

6. Cut the chicken into thick slices then place on a bed of rice with a tablespoon of mango chutney the side.

Spanish Omelet

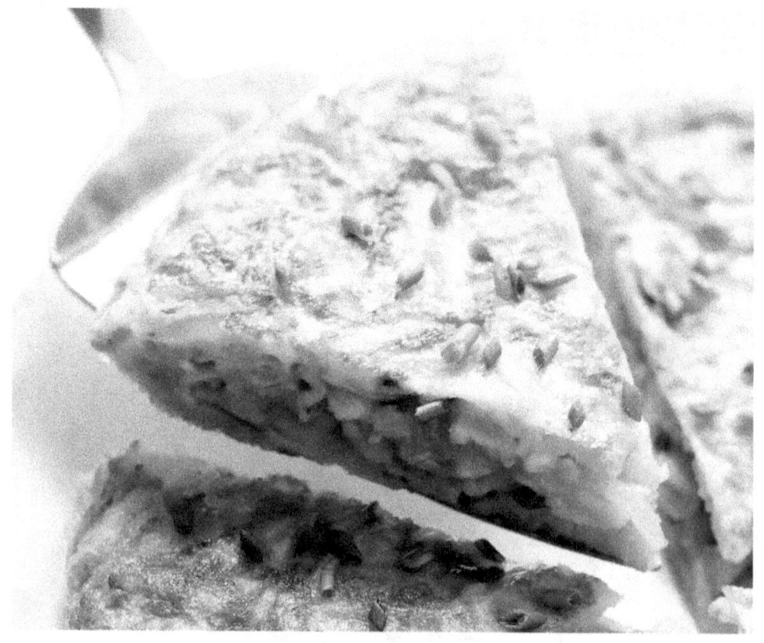

A fluffy vegetarian tortilla. Perfect served hot or cold.

Serves: 2

Time: 22 mins.

Calories per serving: 310

Ingredients:

- Eggs (6)
- Chorizo sausage (2oz, finely chopped)

- Paprika (1 tsp)

- Leaf parsley (1 tbsp, freshly chopped, flat)

- Salt pepper (to taste)

Directions:

1. Join all the ingredients together.

2. Pour the mixture into a shallow, well-greased, dish (steam-proof).

3. Place in the steamer on the bottom tier. Use the lid to cover the steamer and steam for approximately 12 minutes.

4. Cut into wedges (thick) and serve immediately.

Chinese Eggs

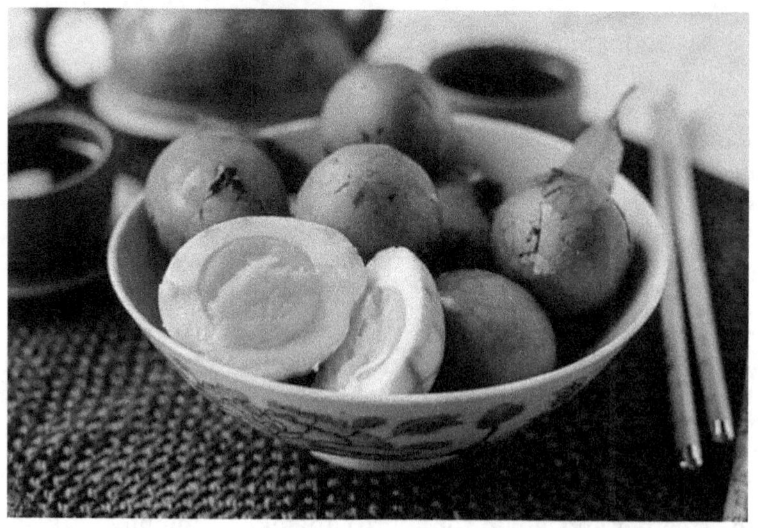

A very simple and interesting breakfast idea.

Serves: 2

Time: 35 mins.

Calories per serving: 120

Ingredients:

- Eggs (3)
- Water (/¾ cup)
- Salt (1 tsp)
- Sesame oil (1 tsp)

- Soy sauce (1 tsp)
- Onions/scallions (4, spring, sliced lengthways)
- Salt pepper (to taste)

Directions:

1. Beat the eggs well and put through a sieve into dish (steam-proof). Add the water salt and mix thoroughly.

2. Allow the mixture stay for a couple minutes. Tightly cover with tin foil and place it in the steamer on the bottom tier.

3. Use the lid to cover the steamer and steam for approximately 20-25 minutes.

4. Embellish with a drop of soy sauce, sesame oil as well as the spring onions (finely chopped).

Spinach Feta Frittata

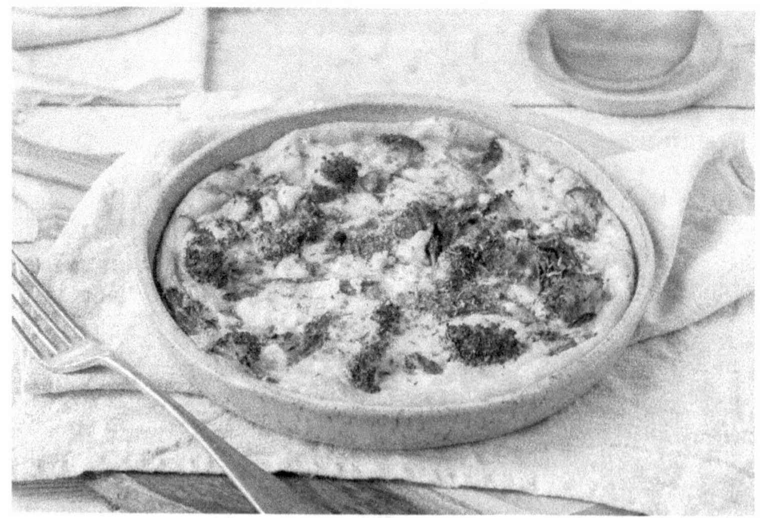

A simple, all-star Spinach and Feta Frittata. Perfect for brunch or weeknight dinner.

Serves: 2

Time: 16 mins.

Calories per serving: 280

Ingredients:

- Eggs (6)
- Spinach (2oz, finely chopped)
- Low fat feta cheese (2oz, crumbled)

- Salt pepper (to taste)

Directions:

1. Join all the ingredients together.

2. Pour the mixture into a shallow, well-greased dish (steam-proof).

3. Place in the steamer on the bottom tier. Use the lid to cover the steamer and steam for approximately 8-12 minutes. Cut into wedges (thick) and serve. Enjoy.

Hardboiled Eggs Prawns

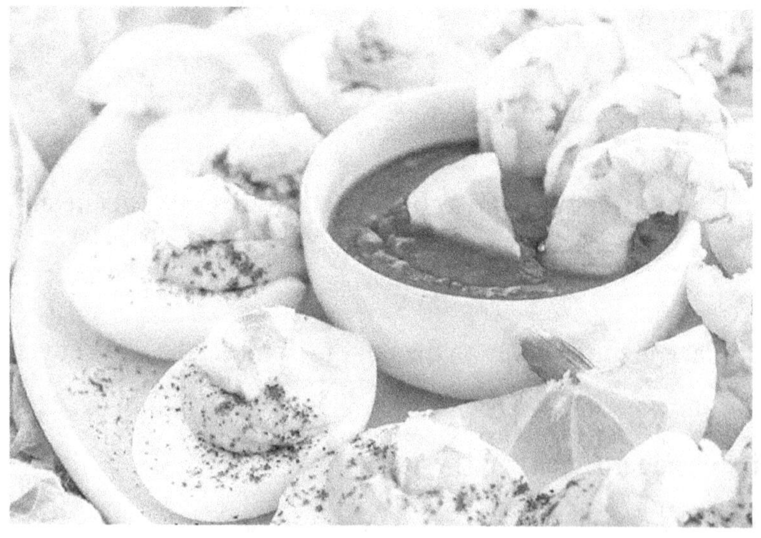

A hearty protein packed recipe. A healthy choice for lunch or light dinner.

Serves: 2

Time: 15 mins.

Calories per serving: 170

Ingredients:

- Eggs (4)
- King prawns (8, large, cooked, peeled)

- Mayonnaise (1 tbsp, low fat)

- Paprika (1 tsp)

- Dill or chives (1 tbsp, chopped)

- Salt pepper (to taste)

Directions:

1. Place the king prawns and eggs into a steamer then boil until eggs are fully hardened and prawns are ready. Transfer to a container filled with ice water and begin to plunge. Peel each egg when they are cool enough.

2. Slice in half (lengthways) then scoop out the yolks. Mash the yolks, mayonnaise and paprika together with a fork.

3. Load the paprika mash back into the egg halves, place a king prawn on top of each (use the mash to secure it) and sprinkle with the dill (chopped).

4. Season with a generous amount salt as well as pepper and serve.

Anchovy Chili Linguine

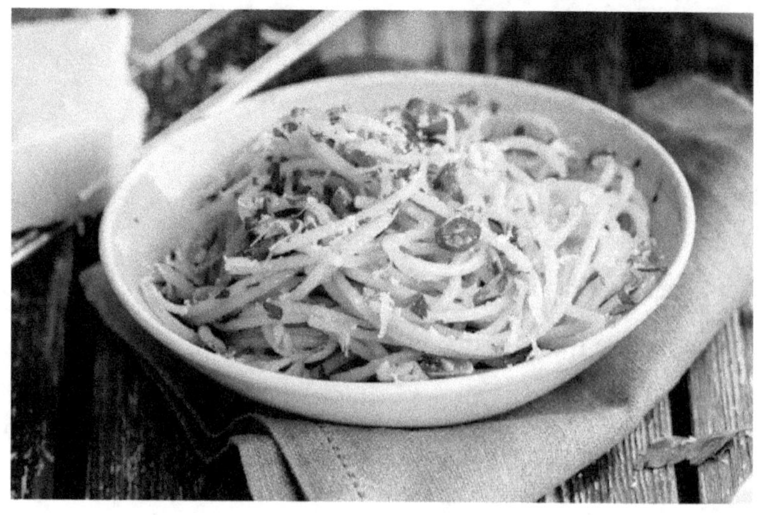

A quick and easy savory dish for your perfect weeknight dinner.

Serves: 2

Time: 30 mins.

Calories per serving: 380

Ingredients:

- Linguine (5oz, snapped in half)
- Salt (Large pinch)
- Anchovy fillets (5, drained)

- Olive oil (2 tbsp)
- Chilies (1 tsp, dried, crushed)
- Garlic cloves (2, peeled)
- Lemon wedges (to serve)
- Salt pepper (to taste)

Directions:

1. In a glass bowl (steam proof) place the pasta and cover using boiling water then add a pinch of salt.

2. When finished, place the bowl into the bottom tier of steamer and use the lid to cover. Steam for a minimum of 5 minutes.

3. While steaming add the oil, anchovy fillets and the chilies (crushed) to a large ramekin dish and place into the bottom tier beside the bowl containing the pasta.

4. Next add the garlic (cloves) to the tier and procced to steam for approximately 10-15 minutes, until pasta is thoroughly cooked, and the garlic until it becomes tender.

5. When time has elapsed begin to drain the pasta and crush the garlic (steamed) and mix well with the anchovy fillets (warm); ensuring that anchovies are broken up properly.

6. Lastly, lightly toss the garlic anchovy oil through the pasta and season and serve using lemon wedges.

Chicken Gyoza

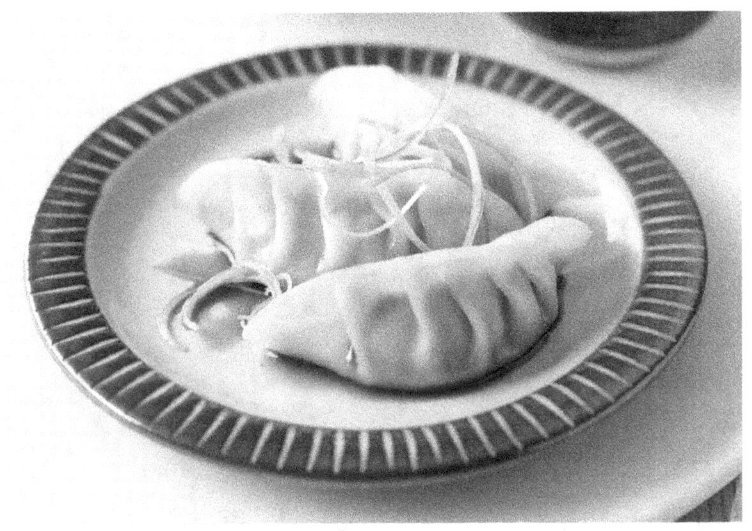

An amazing Chicken Gyoza recipe. Crunchy dumplings on the outside and tender chicken on the inside.

Serves: 2

Time: 25 mins.

Calories per serving: 385

Ingredients:

- Ground chicken (9 oz, ground)
- Cabbage (finely shredded)
- Garlic cloves (2, crushed)

- Ground ginger crushed chili (½ tsp each)
- Oyster sauce (1 tbsp)
- Soy sauce (1 tbsp)
- Salt brown sugar (½ tsp each)
- Gyoza skins (10-12, ready-made)
- Sweet chili dipping sauce (2 tbsp)
- Salt pepper (to taste)

Directions:

1. First step is to place all ingredients into a food processor apart from the sweet chili sauce and dumpling wrapper. Pulse until well combined.

2. Lay out the gyoza skins and place about 2 teaspoons of the chicken mixture into the center of each skin. Use a little water to wet edges then fold over and pinch the newly closed edge to make a little parcel.

3. Place the dumplings in the bottom tier of the steamer. Cover with the lid and steam for 10-12 minutes or until the dumplings are cooked through.

4. Serve with the sweet chili dipping sauce.

Honey Chicken Kebabs

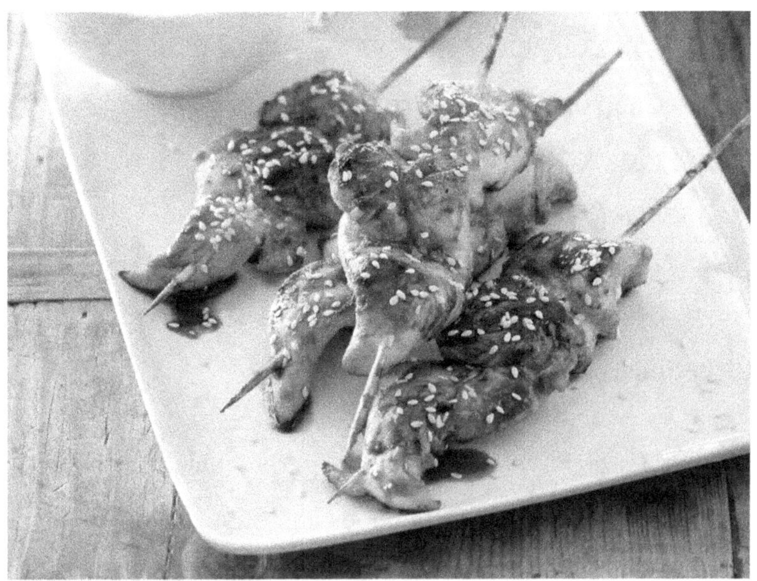

Savory, sweet and sticky chicken on skewers. A favorite of many.

Serves: 2

Time: 25 mins.

Calories per serving: 380

Ingredients:

- Chicken breasts (11 oz, cubed)
- Garlic clove (1, crushed)

- Soy sauce (2 tbsp)

- Clear honey (1 tbsp)

- Olive oil (1 tbsp)

- Cherry tomatoes (7oz)

- Leaf parsley (1 tbsp, freshly chopped, flat)

- Salt pepper (to taste)

- Wooden kebab sticks

Directions:

1. In a large bowl combine the garlic, chicken (cubed), honey, soy sauce, cherry tomatoes and olive oil together.

2. Next, place the freshly coated chicken and cherry tomatoes onto wooden skewers in turn to make a minimum of 4-6 kebabs.

3. Place kebabs on the bottom tier of steamer and use lid to cover. Leave to steam for approximately 10-15 minutes, until chicken is thoroughly cooked.

4. Sprinkle using the parsley (chopped), season and serve. Enjoy.

Fruit Salsa Chicken Rice

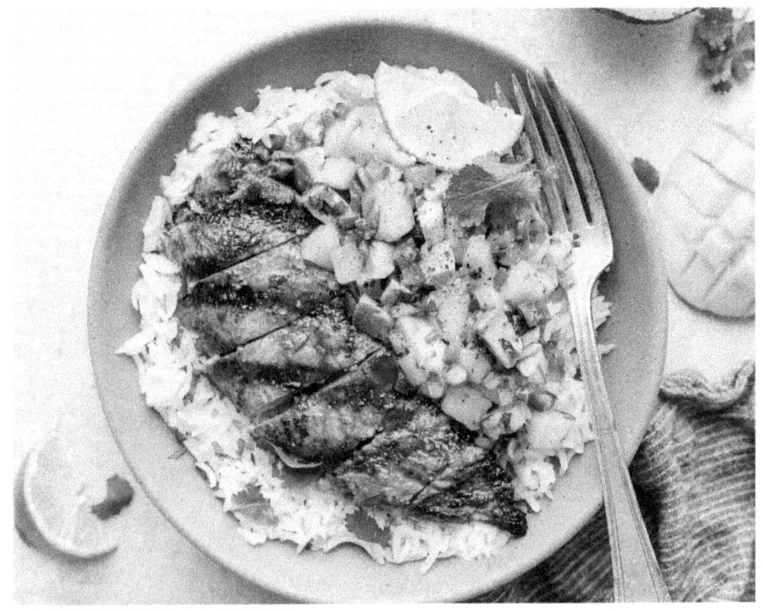

A tropical pineapple salsa with a hint of lime juice adds a nice flair to this quick and easy main dish.

Serves: 2

Time: 50 mins.

Calories per serving: 440

Ingredients:

- Rice (3½ oz, long grain)
- Boiling water (1 cup)
- Salt (Large pinch)
- Chicken breasts (2, 4 oz)
- Coriander/cilantro (1 small bunch, fresh)
- Onions/scallions (1 small bunch, spring)
- Lime juice (1 tbsp)
- Pineapple chunks (7 oz, tinned)
- Salt pepper (to taste)

Directions:

1. In a glass bowl (steam-proof) combine the water, rice and salt then place into the second tier of steamer.

2. Use the lid to cover the steamer and steam for approximately 12-15 minutes.

3. While steaming procced to season the chicken and add the spring onions, fresh coriander, pineapple and lime juice into to a food processor.

4. Blend until a chunky fruit salsa is made. Place salsa into a small dish (steam-proof) and cover using a piece of aluminum foil.

5. Place the salsa dish and the chicken into the bottom tier of steamer and cover using the lid.

6. Steam for approximately 20 minutes, until the chicken is thoroughly cooked.

7. Serve chicken onto a bed of rice with the salsa (hot) poured over the top.

Chicken with Tomato Basil Sauce

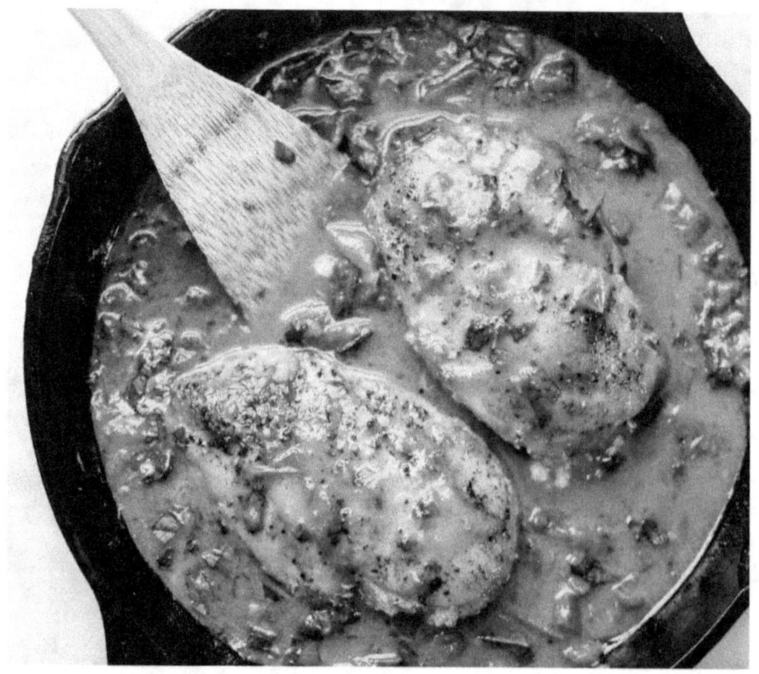

This tasty recipe is quick and easy, well flavored with tomato herbs and basil sauce. A delicious weeknight dinner for family and friends.

Serves: 2

Time: 30 mins.

Calories per serving: 310

Ingredients:

- Chicken breasts (2, 5 oz)
- Garlic clove (1, crushed)
- Tomato ketchup (4 tbsp)
- Basil (large bunch, fresh)
- Cherry tomatoes (11 oz)
- Watercress (5 oz)
- Salt pepper (to taste)

Directions:

1. First step is to season the chicken. Then add the ketchup, basil, garlic clove, and the tomatoes into a food processor.

2. Pulse for approximately 10-30 seconds until a chunky sauce is made.

3. Transfer the sauce from the processor and place into a dish (steam-proof) covered with aluminum foil.

4. Place the chicken breasts into the bottom tier of steamer and the sauce dish into the second tier.

5. Use lid to cover steamer and steam for approximately 20 minutes, until the chicken is thoroughly.

6. Transfer chicken breasts to a plate and pour over the tomato sauce and serve with the watercress on the side.

Lime Squid Salad

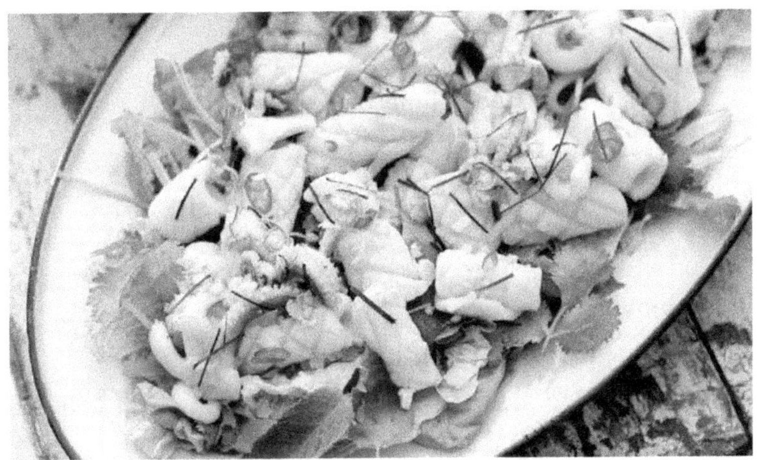

This delectable recipe is quick and easy to prepare with a surprisingly low caloric value.

Serves: 2

Time: 16 mins.

Calories per serving: 220

Ingredients:

- Prepared squid (11oz, cut into rings)
- Red chili (1, deseeded finely chopped)
- Garlic cloves (2, crushed)
- Fish sauce (1 tbsp)

- Lime juice (1 tbsp)

- Soy sauce (1 tbsp)

- Brown sugar (½ tsp)

- Romaine lettuce (1, shredded)

- Cherry tomatoes (5oz, halved)

- Salt pepper (to taste)

Directions:

1. First step is to season the squid. When finished, add the garlic, chili (chopped) fish sauce, soy sauce, lime juice, and sugar into a ramekin dish.

2. Use a piece of aluminum foil to cover and transfer to the bottom tier of steamer along with the squid rings.

3. Cover steamer using the lid and steam for approximately 4-6 minutes, until the squid is thoroughly cooked.

4. Serve squid on a bed of tomatoes and lettuce (shredded) lettuce with the lime dressing (hot) poured over the top.

Lime Ginger Baby Carrots

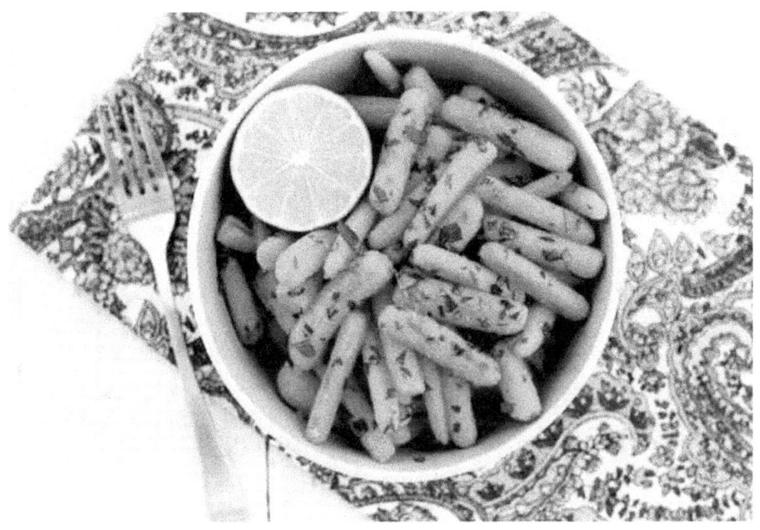

This delicious recipe is prepared in less than an hour and is packed with many essential vitamins and minerals.

Serves: 2

Time: 35 mins.

Calories per serving: 80

Ingredients:

- Baby carrots (7 oz, fresh)
- Butter (1oz, spread, low fat)
- Ginger (1 tsp, freshly grated)

- Garlic clove (1, crushed)
- Lime juice (2 tsp)
- Salt (large pinch)
- Salt pepper (to taste)

Directions:

1. First step is to scrub carrots and transfer to the bottom tier of steamer.

2. Cover using the lid and steam for approximately 8-10 minutes.

3. When finished, add the ginger, butter, garlic, salt and lime juice to a ramekin dish. Cover dish tightly using a piece of aluminum foil and place on a tier above the carrots (steaming).

4. Cover steamer once more using the lid and continue steaming the carrots for an additional 15 minutes, until carrots are thoroughly cooked and becomes tender. When finished, place in a bowl and pour over the butter (melted) and combine well until the carrots are coated evenly.

5. Season and serve. Enjoy.

Steamed Bananas

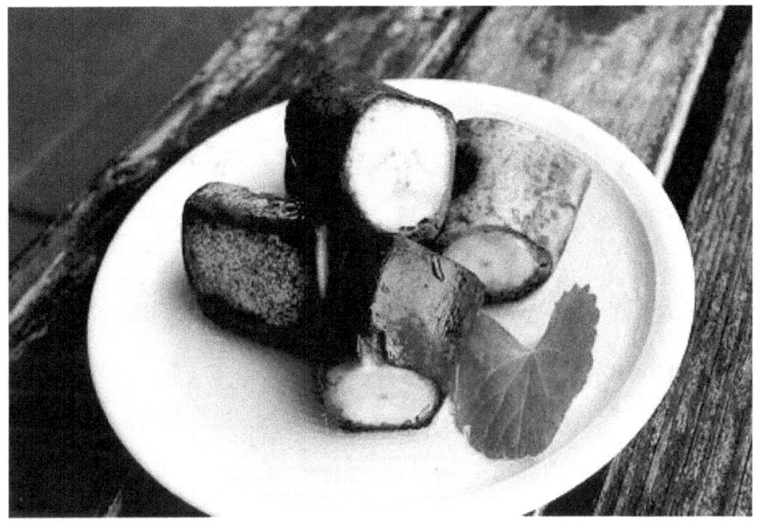

An exotic recipe utilizing hot steamy bananas.

Serves: 2

Time: 20 mins.

Calories per serving: 140

Ingredients:

- Bananas (2, large)
- Honey (2 tsp, clear)
- coconut cream (1 tbsp)

Directions:

1. First step is to remove the both ends from the bananas and transfer to the bottom tier of steamer.

2. Steam for approximately15 minutes, until banana skins become blackened.

3. Drizzle bananas using honey and serve with coconut cream (dollop).

Simple Mexican Corn

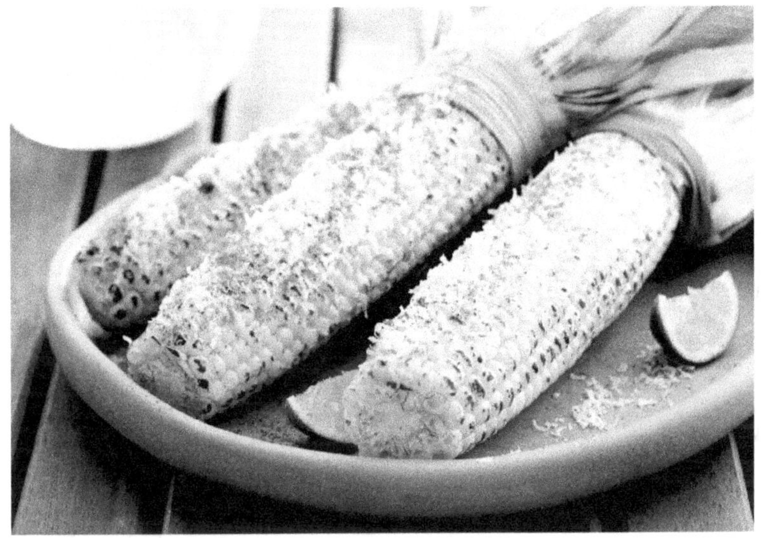

This delicious and steamy corn recipe is a sure crowd pleaser.

Serves: 2

Time: 35 mins.

Calories per serving: 200

Ingredients:

- Corn on the cob (2, fresh, medium)
- Extra virgin olive oil (1 tbsp)

- Paprika (2 tsp)
- Lime juice (2 tsp)
- Salt pepper (to taste)

Directions:

1. First step is to separate the silky husks from the corn then place the cobs into steamer on the bottom tier.

2. Cover using lid and steam for approximately 30 minutes, until the corn (fresh) becomes tender.

3. When finished, Combine both the olive oil, paprika and lime juice together.

4. Once corn becomes tender transfer to a bowl and brush using spiced oil.

5. Season well and serve. Enjoy.

Cheese Chive Omelet

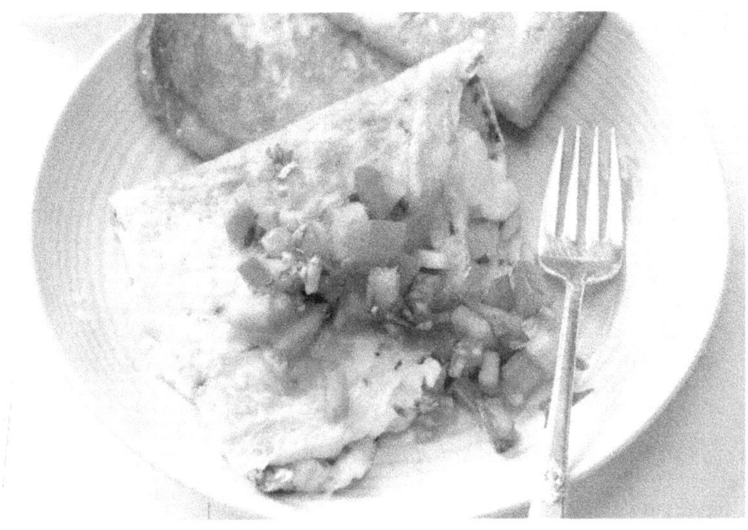

Just one bite of this herbaceous creamy omelet will leave you speechless.

Serves: 2

Time: 15 mins.

Calories per serving: 170

Ingredients:

- Eggs (4)
- Low fat (2oz, grated, cheddar cheese)
- Chopped chives (4 tbsp)

- Salt pepper (to taste)

Directions:

1. Put all the ingredients together.

2. Separate the mixture equally between two lightly greased, shallow, dishes (steam-proof).

3. Place on both the first and second tier of the steamer.

4. Use the lid and steam for 10 minutes. Fold omelets in half and serve immediately.

Conclusion

Congrats on cooking your way through all 30 delicious steam recipes that are hassle-free and delicious. The next step from here would be to continue practicing. With every single steam recipe, you create you will see magic being created.

After you have accomplished that, come on back over and find another amazing journey to partake in from cuisines across the globe in another one of our books. We hope to see you again soon.

Happy cooking!